Intermittent Fasting

The Ultimate Beginner's Guide To The Intermittent Fasting Diet Lifestyle - Delay, Don't Deny Food - Finally Lose Weight, Burn Fat, Live A Healthier & More Productive Life

By Simone Jacobs

For more great books visit:

HMWPublishing.com

Get another book for Free

I want to thank you for purchasing this book and offer you another book (just as long and valuable as this book), "Health & Fitness Mistakes You Don't Know You're Making", completely free.

Visit the link below to signup and receive it:

www.hmwpublishing.com/gift

In this book, I will break down the most common health & fitness mistakes, you are probably committing right now, and I will reveal how you can easily get in the best shape of your life!

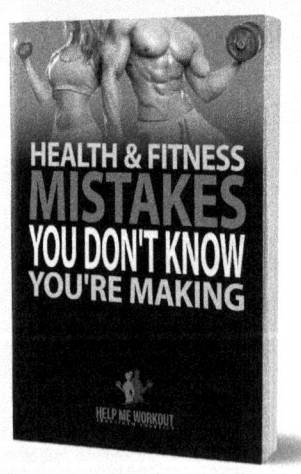

In addition to this valuable gift, you will also have an opportunity to get our new books for free, enter giveaways, and receive other valuable emails from me. Again, visit the link to sign up:

www.hmwpublishing.com/gift

Table of Contents

Chapter 1: Lose Weight and Build Muscle on a Time-Tested, Ancient Healing Tradition 4

Gear Your Body, Mind, and Spirit towards Healing and Weight Loss 5
    A Brief Glance at the History of Fasting 6
    Modern-Day Fasting 7
    Fasting is not Starving 8
Teach Your Body to Burn Glucose and Fat 9
    Recalibrating a System Dependent on Food ... 9
    Make Your Body into a Sugar-and-Fat-Burning Machine 11
Fasting is the Easiest Way to be Healthy 15

Chapter 2: The Virtues of Intermittent Fasting 19

    Decrease Insulin Levels 21
    Boost Weight Loss 22
    Burn Belly Fat Faster 23
    Stimulate the Production of Growth Hormone ... 24
    Increase Adrenaline Levels 26
    Regulates Functions of Cells, Hormones, and Genes 27
        Repair Cells 28
        Alters Gene Expression 28
        Relieve Inflammation 29
        Develop Strong Heart 29
        Anti-Aging 30

Improve Your Focus and Mental Clarity 31
Release Energy for Healing................................33
Fosters Spiritual Growth 35
Reasons Why Fasting Works...............................36
    Relaxing...36
    Lengthens Life Span 37
    Complement Chemo Therapy.......................37

Chapter 3: Effectively Adapting to the Healthy Change 40

Electrolyte Deficiency..40
Uric Acid Elevation..42
After-Fast Weight Gain 43
Lean Muscle Mass Loss.......................................45
Not Everyone Can Fast..46
    Those Who Shouldn't Fast.............................47
Fasting for Women..48
Intermittent Fasting Options for Women............49
    Crescendo Method 50

Chapter 4: Listen to the Needs of Your Body 55

Buffer Your Weight Loss and Muscle Gain Journey 55
Start Your Diet with a 1-Day Fruit or Juice Fast .56
#1 - Leangains Method (16:8 Fasting).................57
#2 - Eat Stop Eat (24-Hour Fasting) 59
#3 - The Warrior Diet (20/4 Diet).......................61
#4 – Fat Loss Forever 63
#5 - UpDayDownDay (Alternate-Day Fasting) ...64

#6 –Fast Diet (5:2 Fasting) 66
#7 – Daniel Fast 67

Chapter 5: Successfully Transitioning into a Healthier You 69

Prepare for the Detoxification and Ketosis Symptoms
.... 69
- Disrupted Sleep Patterns and Fatigue 70
- Headache 70
- Nausea 71
- Cravings and Hunger 71

Stay Hydrated 72
Prefer Overnight Fasting 72
Transform Your Thinking Process 72
Start When You're Busy 73
Hit the Gym 73

Conclusion 76

Final Words 78

About the Co-Author 79

Introduction

Do you have a weight loss problem? Do you continuously watch out for answers in the market hoping for a quick and efficient solution to your problem? If you do, then this book is entirely right for you!

Everyone seems to be in a rush searching for ways to weight loss nowadays. A myriad of offers covering dieting, health and food supplements, physical fitness programs, and various training workshops are flooding the entire health and fitness market. All these entail costs and effort on your part and mostly turn out to be not as effective as these marketers promised in their glamorous ads.

However, there's an ongoing solution that many are resorting to nowadays. Although it is not exempted from cynic opinions, it is a lot better than those options being offered in the market. For one, it does not require your extra effort to do it, and it does not hit your pocket like it does when you prepare for a new set of diet or enrol in a physical fitness program.

The popularity of intermittent fasting is gaining momentum in the market today when people are getting tired of numerous diets that sound easy to do at the first attempt but usually do not work well in the long run.

This book, "***Intermittent Fasting: 7 Beginner's Intermittent Fasting Methods for Women & Men- Weight loss and Build Lean Muscle Hacks***" is designed to provide you with an efficient alternative solution to your problem regarding weight.

This book will further enlighten you about the fundamentals of Intermittent Fasting and how it proves to be the coolest, quickest, and easiest way to lose weight while building lean muscles for both men and women. Grab a copy of this book before it's gone and start dropping pounds in fewer days!

Also, before you get started, I recommend you <u>joining our email newsletter</u> to receive updates on any upcoming new book releases or promotions. You can sign-up for free, and as a bonus, you will receive a free gift. Our "*Health & Fitness Mistakes You Don't Know You're Making*" book! This book has been written to demystify, expose the top do's and don'ts and to finally equip you with the information you need to get in the best shape of your life. Due to the overwhelming amount of mis-information and lies told by magazines and self-proclaimed "gurus", it's becoming harder and harder to get reliable information to get in shape. As opposed to having to go through dozens of biased, unreliable and un-trustworthy sources to get your health & fitness information. Everything you need to help you has been broken down in this book for you to easily follow and to immediately get results to achieve your desired fitness goals in the shortest amount of time.

Once again, to join our free email newsletter and to receive a free copy of this valuable book, please visit the link and signup now: www.hmwpublishing.com/gift

Chapter 1: Lose Weight and Build Muscle on a Time-Tested, Ancient Healing Tradition

The demands and responsibilities of life often lead to various health problems, especially when you are too distracted and you overlook the importance and the practice of a healthy lifestyle and eating habit. More often than not, you do notice the slow changes happening to your body, but you are too busy to do anything about it. The only time you will ever really decide to do something about your concern is when you are already getting sick to the point that you cannot work efficiently.

So your search for solutions begins, but which diet, training, and health fitness program REALLY works? There are tons and tons of them out there. The answer is simple. Teach your body to heal itself and to lose weight by learning when to eat and when to stop eating.

Gear Your Body, Mind, and Spirit towards Healing and Weight Loss

Learning when to eat and when to stop eating is a practice called Intermittent Fasting (IF). This concept is nothing new. It's a method used by many people all over the world since time immemorial. Humans go through long periods without eating for most of our history for various religious reasons and when the food source is scarce. In fact, when we sleep, we inadvertently fast.

We fast when we sleep? Yes, indeed! If you typically eat your dinner by 8 pm and have your breakfast at 8 am the morning you wake up, you are fasting for 12 hours and eating for 12 hours. We call this fasting method as a 12/12 fast. Isn't that great news? You can fast while sleeping! I mean it's no effort at all if you choose to practice this method.

But fasting is not exclusive to humans, even animals fast when they are ill or stressed, and sometimes when they feel slightly uneasy. Fasting is a natural tendency for every organism, whether animal or human, to conserve energy during critical times and to seek balance and to rest.

A Brief Glance at the History of Fasting

Hippocrates, Galen, Socrates, Plato, and Aristotle, as well as early great healers, thinkers, and other philosophers all praised the benefits of fasting for healing and health therapy. Paracelsus, one of the three fathers of Western medicine said, "Fasting is the greatest remedy--the physician within."

Early spiritual and religious groups fast as part of their rites and ceremonies, especially during the fall and spring equinoxes. Almost every dominant religion observe fasting for various spiritual benefits.

North and South American Indian traditions, Hinduism, Buddhism, Islam, Gnosticism, Judaism, and Christianity use one form of fasting or another for sacrifice or mourning, penance, spiritual vision, or purification.

Yogic practices, including fasting, date as far back as back as thousands of years. Paramahansa Yogananda, a famous yogi and guru said, "Fasting is a natural method of healing." Likewise, Ayurveda, ancient healing practice, includes fasting as part of its therapy.

However, scientific medicine became dominant and developed better drugs. Fasting and other Naturopathic ways of healing fell off the stage. Recently, many people searching for health solutions return to the old ways.

Modern-Day Fasting

The time-tested, ancient healing tradition of intermittent fasting is back in the spotlight and gaining popularity among many people today. Between 1895-1985, Herbert Shelton, a physician, followed and supervised the fasts of over 40,000 people. During the century and concluded that fasting is a radical and fundamental process that is older than any practice of healing the body, an instinctive method when an organism is sick.

Even though IF is a practice that is as old as the human race itself, modern science and recent studies now reveal that knowing when and eat and when to stop eating creates significant positive changes in the body, resetting the entire system that increases its ability to function at high levels both mentally and physically. Indeed, many research supports the health benefits of IF.

Food abstinence keeps the mind and memory sharp, reduces the risk of various diseases, and keeps the body cells healthy. A study titled, "The Scientific Evidence Surrounding Intermittent Fasting" conducted by Amber Simmons, Ph.D., pointed out that IF together with caloric restriction, is an effective method to promote weight loss in obese and overweight individuals.

Fasting is not Starving

When people hear the word fasting, they often think of it as synonymous to starving. This misconception can often lead people astray and choose other never-been-heard, exotic, and sometimes complicated, diet method.

Starving is when you don't know when your next meal will come. On the other hand, fasting is a practice where you strategically plan periods of when to 'eat' and 'stop eating.' In fact, the word breakfast is the meal you eat to break the fast that you do every day while you are sleeping.

Moreover, it is not the fasting but the caloric restriction that comes with limiting what you eat that produces the health benefits. For example, if you eat at 6 am in the morning and refrain from eating anything within the next 9 hours, then you are actually restricting your calorie without counting, given that you only eat the right amount of food and do not eat double servings of your meal at breakfast. The key to IF is 'discipline,' not starvation.

Teach Your Body to Burn Glucose and Fat

Intermittent Fasting is not a diet per se, but a method in which you teach your body to compartmentalize into "eating" and "fasting" periods. How does learning when to eat and when not to eat help a person lose weight?

Recalibrating a System Dependent on Food

The body metabolizes fat and glucose from the food you eat as its primary source of energy. Carbohydrates are the primary source of glucose. When you eat carb-rich diet, they are broken down into the simpler form called glucose. This substance circulates freely in the bloodstream into every cell of your body as the energy source. When you eat, you supply your body with enough glucose to sustain your body with enough energy to run for 3-4 hours.

Excess glucose goes to the liver and muscles for storage and becomes the body's secondary source of energy. When the cells run out of free circulating blood glucose, the body will break down and metabolize the stored glycogen and transforms it into glucose. Glycogen is the reason you do not have to eat every 15 to 20 minutes. In fact, glycogen stores in your body can sustain you for 6 up to 24 hours after your last meal.

The problem begins when you consume excessive amounts of carbohydrates. Your body runs out of storage capacity for glycogen, so the liver converts it into adipose tissue, triglycerides, or fat for long-term storage. And because you continuously supply the body with energy by eating 3 meals and 2 to 3 snacks in between, the cells consistently have an excess supply of glucose, which is converted into more glycogen in the liver and fat in the body.

Do you see the picture clearer now? Most of us consume more energy than our body can utilize, so the system stores them as glycogen and body fat. We also tend to eat when we feel slightly hungry, so we do not give our cells the chance to use these stored fuels. Thus, we end up adding more and more stored glycogen and adipose tissue into our system, which leads to various health problems, including diabetes, overweight, and other related illnesses linked to high-sugar and high-fat content in the body.

Moreover, when we eat continuously, your body is used to the constant supply of free-circulating glucose, which could lead to insulin resistance. It is a condition where the body is repeatedly with high levels of sugar and insulin in the blood until your system no longer produces sufficient insulin to metabolize glucose or become resistant to its effect.

Make Your Body into a Sugar-and-Fat-Burning Machine

The simple principle behind intermittent fasting is "discipline." **Not feeding or eating for periods gives the body a chance to burn off excess and stored glucose and fat. Practicing IF recalibrates your body** from a system that is dependent on food into a sugar-and-fat-burning machine.

The human body is a fantastic mechanism with a developed system that allows it to deal with periods of low food source. It undergoes the 5 sequent process or stages below to sustain the need for energy.

Feeding

Eating food raises the insulin levels of the body, allowing the tissues of the body to utilize the glucose as energy. During this stage, the liver stores it any excess as glycogen within itself. When the storage space of glycogen in the liver is full, the organ transforms the surplus it into triglyceride or fat for extended storage.

Glycogen Breakdown

Within 6 to 24 hours after your meal, the insulin level will start to fall. During this period, the body will begin metabolizing the stored glycogen as energy and this secondary source of glucose in the liver can sustain the body for about 24 hours.

Gluconeogenesis

After roughly 24 hours up to 2 days without a ready source of glucose, the body utilizes amino acids, the simple form of protein, to manufacture new glucose during the process called "gluconeogenesis." In a non-diabetic person, the glucose levels will fall but stay within the normal range.

Ketosis

After 2 to 3 days without food, the low insulin levels in the body stimulates the breakdown of triglycerides or stored fat for energy during the process called lipolysis. The body metabolizes the stored fat into 3-fatty acid chains and glycerol backbone. The body uses the glycerol for gluconeogenesis or manufacturing of new glucose. The body tissues can readily utilize the 3-fatty acid chains as energy.

However, the brain cannot, so the body metabolizes the 3-fatty acid chains into ketone bodies or energy that can pass in the blood-brain barrier as the brain's fuel source, which is mainly in the forms of acetoacetate and beta-hydroxybutyrate, to sustain the brain's energy needs.

Four days after the body's last meal, 75 percent of the energy used by your mind is from ketones, and the amount increases over 70 times during the fasting period.

Protein conservation

On the 5th day, fasting stimulates the production of growth hormone to help the body maintain lean tissue and muscle mass. During this period, the metabolic system utilizes ketones and fatty acids entirely as the source of energy. The level of adrenaline (norepinephrine) also increases to adapt to the change, giving the body more fuel.

Of course, you will not be depriving yourself of food nor be starving during intermittent fasting. As mentioned, IF practice focuses on scheduling when to eat and when not to feed, which gradually teaches the body to utilize excess and stored sugar and fat as energy instead of relying on food. This traditional method opens the gates to better health, weight loss, and building of muscle mass and lean tissue.

Fasting is the Easiest Way to be Healthy

The best thing about intermittent fasting is you can incorporate it into any healthy and balanced diet. When diet is particularly hard to follow, you have the option to stop worrying about what to eat at the very least. It is also convenient when you do not have to prepare meals for a period. Plus, you can save on some amount of money, too. But that's not the real reason why most people love intermittent fasting. There is more to the practicality IF practice offers.

Some people developed the habit of not eating healthy food choices and unhealthy feeding patterns throughout their lifetime, including eating in between meals, choosing fast and junk foods over a well-balanced diet, or just routinely giving in to constant food cravings when they feel hungry. All these constitute an unhealthy lifestyle, which can eventually lead to serious health problems.

Going on a diet and doing a fasting practice both leads to weight loss; hence, people aiming to shed their excess fat face a predicament when choosing which method to adapt to a healthier lifestyle.

According to Dr. Michael Eades, co-author of the famous book, "Protein Power," it is always easy to contemplate on a diet, but it is often harder to execute. Contrary to an eating program, intermittent fasting is just the opposite, it appears to be too hard to contemplate, but once you perform, you find it is not that hard at all.

Going on a diet is always easier during the first few days, but the longer you stay on it, you find it less and less appealing. The reason why most diets do not work out in the long run. Only a few people manage to integrate one form of eating into their lifestyle.

Thinking of fasting would always send you to believe you can't survive a day without eating, especially for those who badly need to fast. However, you will find it easier to do when you start doing it. Turning it into a habit and making it a part of your lifestyle is easier done than just contemplating on it. It's hard to overcome the idea of not eating, but once you go over the hurdle, intermittent fasting is, in fact, easier to do than following a diet.

Intermittent fasting acts as a reset button. It does not regulate nor does not tell you what kind of food you should eat and not consume. Instead, it determines the best time when you should have a proper, healthy, and well-balanced meal. It's an eating pattern that you integrate into your lifestyle to recalibrate your body and improve your health.

Key Takeaways:

- Fasting is a time-tested, ancient healing tradition that can help you lose weight and build muscles.

- The practice of scheduling your feeding time gears your body, mind, and spirit towards various health benefits.

- The key of intermittent fasting is discipline, not starving. It is simply planning when to eat and when not to eat.

- Fasting with caloric restriction recalibrates your body from a sugar-fueled system into a fat-burning machine.

- It resets the button, giving your body the chance to relax and direct energy for healing, weight loss, and muscle building.

Chapter 2: The Virtues of Intermittent Fasting

Before you start fasting, you need to understand what hormonal adaptation your body will undergo concerning fat loss, so you do not immediately plunge into it just to stop before it even starts working on your body.

For starters, let's review the "fed state" and the "fasted state" of the human body. A human body is in a fed state when it is taking in and digesting food. Generally, the feeding starts at the time you start eating the food, and this will last for 3-5 hours while your digestive system is working on it.

While in the fed state, your body cannot burn fat efficiently because of the high level of insulin in the body that enables the sugar to be utilized by the cells as energy.

However, after the digestion process, your body will soon be in the post-absorptive state, which means that your body is no longer working on processing a meal. This period will last from 8 to 12 hours after your last meal, and during this period, your body starts to gain entry to the fasted state. It is during this time that your body begins to burn fat, and your insulin level will begin to lower.

Take note that your body only enters the fasted state 12 hours after your last meal, and since most of us eat 3-6 meals a day, it is rare that your body is getting into this condition; hence, you are depriving your body of experiencing the fat-burning state.

The reason why those who are practicing IF were able to lose fat even without changing the kind and the quantity of food they are eating or how often they have their exercise. Intermittent fasting allows your body to undergo the fat-burning process that you rarely experience when you have your regular eating schedule.

Intermittent fasting maximizes the glycogen and fat-burning mechanism of the body. During the "fasting state," your system undergoes various hormonal adaptations that lead to weight loss and muscle gain.

Decrease Insulin Levels

All food raises the insulin levels in the body. Therefore, the most consistent, efficient, and effective strategy for lowering it is to avoid foods. If you are a non-diabetic person, your blood glucose levels remain normal as your body starts to switch into fat burning. This adaptation is evident in as short as 24-36 hours of fasting. The longer you fast, the longer the duration of reduced insulin and the decrease is more significant.

According to a study titled, "Alternate-day fasting in nonobese subjects: effects on body weight, body composition, and energy metabolism," fasting every other day is an effective method to reduce insulin levels without affecting the normal glucose levels of the body.

Fasting decreases insulin level by 20-31 percent and lowers your blood sugar by 3-6% once your body utilizes stored fat starts as fuel in place of carbohydrates, thus, likewise reducing the risk for Type 2 diabetes.

Boost Weight Loss

Another reason why intermittent fasting is popular these days is that scientific studies prove it is a powerful technique for weight loss. We love to eat food rich in carbohydrates and fats, and then we panic once we see our weight measurement rise.

With an IF practice, you can choose between eating fewer meals or entirely not consume any food for a few days. This process is sure to reduce the overall calorie intake, as well as normalize the hormonal change that inhibits fat burning as it triggers the release of norepinephrine (noradrenaline).

Through short-term fasting, you can increase your metabolic rate up to 14 percent. Intermittent fasting likewise results in weight loss by changing your caloric equation, e.g., taking in fewer calories and burning more of it.

The same study that showed the effects of alternate-day fasting in reducing insulin levels further revealed after 22 days, the 16 people who ate every other day lost 2.5 percent of their body weight.

The study further showed that their hunger increased during the first fasting day and remained high. There was no significant change in their resting metabolic rate (RMR) and respiratory quotient (RQ) from day 1 to day 21, but on the 22nd day, their RQ decreased, which resulted in a significant increase in fat oxidation or loss in their bodies up to 15 grams and more.

However, since hunger on fasting days did not decrease, the authors of the research suggested that eating a small meal during fasting days make this approach more acceptable. Nevertheless, the study corroborated that fasting is an efficient and fast strategy to lose excess weight.

Burn Belly Fat Faster

Belly fat or what we call the "love handles" are the most dangerous of all the fats stored in your body. The name may sound appealing, but love handles are very sinister. They are hazardous visceral fats that tend to build around the internal organs and later lead to severe illnesses.

However, a study revealed that undergoing intermittent fasting not only reduce body weight; it also decreases waist circumference by 4 to 7 percent.

Stimulate the Production of Growth Hormone

Growth hormone (HG) or somatotropin or human growth hormone (HGH or hGH) stimulates cell reproduction and regeneration and growth, thus, is very vital to human development. It is a natural hormone produced by the pituitary gland, and the majority of the secretion occurs during sleep. As you age the level of HG production declines and it can lead to decreased lean muscle mass, lack of energy, and increase in body fat.

The relationship between human growth hormone and insulin is a complicated one. HGH is the antagonist of the latter and vice versa. When you have insulin resistance, your body continually has high amounts of insulin to balance the high volume of glucose in your body, which decreases the production of GH.

On the other hand, insulin resistance may be the result of HGH deficiency. When your body produces high levels of growth hormone, it competes with the same receptor sites as insulin and instead of metabolizing glucose as the source of energy, the cells burn fat instead. Insulin production decreases and the system cannot adequately stabilize the high amount of sugar in the body. Moreover, people with decreased HGH tend to have excessive body fat content. They also have reduced exercise tolerance and muscle strength.

The fed state inhibits HGH secretion since the body raises the levels of insulin to metabolize the glucose from your food as the source of energy when you eat. Fasting for as little as 5 days increases the secretion of human growth hormone by up to 2 times. When you are fasting, you are decreasing the supply of glucose in the body, which reduces the production of insulin. When the amount of insulin in the body is low, the amount of GHG increases to adapt to the change, burning fat for the energy it needs and losing weight in the process.

Increase growth hormone levels in the body raise the amounts of circulating insulin-like growth factor I (IGF-I), which also regulate growth. The increase of both GHG and IGF-I results in the growth of muscle mass, as well as increase muscle strength.

Increase Adrenaline Levels

Our body is equipped with a survival mechanism that triggers it to go into a survival mode when you are hungry or tired. So when it becomes desperate, the body enhances this instinct so you can have more energy to move and hunt for food.

When you are fasting, your body experiences mild stress that boosts adrenaline production. It is similar to how your body responses when you are exercising or when a dog chases you on the way home. Your natural fight-or-flight hormone kicks in to ensure your safety or survival during dangerous occurrences. Generally, the higher the stress, the higher the adrenaline secretion occurs.

Intermittent fasting is a great way to put your body under stress without actually putting yourself in danger. As your cells start to utilize fat as the source of energy, it signals the body that you need to forage – a primitive instinct that allows early humans to hunt and search for food during times source is scarce, ensuring survival.

Practicing IF naturally stimulates adrenaline secretion, which unlocks and utilizes stored energy – muscle glycogen and fat. Simply put, adrenaline promotes the release of stored glucose from its locations in the body, increasing metabolism even during rested state. Moreover, increased adrenaline levels boost concentration, focus, and energy.

Regulates Functions of Cells, Hormones, and Genes

Once you are in the fasted state, your body initiates repair of cells and regulates your hormone levels to have your body fat working. Here are examples of some changes that occur while you are fasting.

Repair Cells

The body induces some cellular repair, like removing toxins and wastes from your body, in a process known as autophagy, which involves breaking down dysfunctional proteins that have built-up inside the cells over time. Increased autophagy can provide your body protection against several diseases, including cancer and Alzheimer's disease.

Alters Gene Expression

A study titled "The effects of fasting on the physiological status and gene expression; an overview" revealed that calorie restriction through reduction of food or eliminating food and caloric beverages for a period changes various signaling pathways and the expression of different genes, leading to longer lifespan and high immunity against diseases.

Moreover, another study revealed that alternate day fasting increased the expression or SIRT1, a gene linked to longevity. Also, another study showed that gene expression in adipogenesis in mice was also altered, leading to faster regulation of reserved triacylglycerol into fuel.

Relieve Inflammation

Researchers disclosed through studies that intermittent fasting shows a significant reduction in inflammation, which is a crucial determinant for many chronic illnesses. A study titled "Ghrelin gene products in acute and chronic inflammation" showed that reducing food and caloric intake increases the production of ghrelin or the hunger hormone, which suppress chronic and acute inflammation, as well as autoimmunity. Low levels of fat tissue also favor the production of anti-inflammatory proteins.

Develop Strong Heart

Intermittent fasting reduces risk factors for heart diseases, including inflammatory markers, blood triglycerides, LDL cholesterol, blood sugar and insulin resistance. A study titled, "Fasting-induced changes in the expression of genes controlling substrate metabolism in the rat heart" revealed that during IF the heart adapts to the changes in glucose and fatty acid metabolism by altering the cardiac energy production at the level of gene expression. This effect reduces fatty acids in the heart.

Moreover, "Intermittent fasting: the next big weight loss fad" stated that IF produce similar effects as intense exercise, heart rate variability while reducing resting heart rate and blood pressure.

Anti-Aging

When tested in rats, intermittent fasting had extended the animal's lifespan by about 83 percent longer. "Intermittent fasting: the next big weight loss fad" revealed that reducing calorie intake in most animals increased lifespan by up to 30 percent. "Dietary restriction in cerebral bioenergetics and redox state" showed that IF delays the appearance of aging markers.

Moreover, "Caloric restriction (CF) and intermittent fasting: Two potential diets for successful brain aging" pointed out that CF and IF practice affects oxygen radical and energy metabolism, as well as systemic cellular stress response, in a manner that protects that neurons against environmental and genetic factors related to aging.

Improve Your Focus and Mental Clarity

As mentioned earlier, fasting stimulates adrenaline secretion that help boosts concentration, focus, and energy. In Chapter 1: Diet on a Time-Tested, Ancient Healing, we also tackled ketones and how fasting the assists the body achieve ketosis, making it a fat-burning machine. During ketosis, the liver breaks down fatty acids into ketones as energy.

Ketones are more efficient fuel for the brain than glucose. When your body burns fuel, either ketones or glucose, it converts it into adenosine triphosphate (ATP), the substance that your cells use as energy. Ketones help produce and increase ATP production better than glucose, creating more energy for the body and the brain to use, thus improving mental performance.

Moreover, other research shows that ketones can process gamma-Aminobutyric acid (GABA) more efficiently. GABA is a molecule that reduces brain stimulation.

When you are not fasting, the body utilizes glucose as its primary source of energy and the brain uses glutamic acid and glutamate for fuel, molecules that stimulate brain function. However, when the brain utilizes the glutamic acid and glutamate as fuel, there is little of the two molecules left to process GABA. Your mind starts to over process without a way to reduce the stimulation, your brain neurons are overstimulated and work excessively, which lead to brain fog or what is known as the inability to recall information or focus on a task. Simply put, too much glutamate means too much brain excitement, which results in brain neurotoxicity, which in some cases lead to seizures, as well as various neurological disorders, such as dementia, amyotrophic lateral sclerosis (ALS), migraines, bipolar disorder, and even depression.

When you are fasting, you give the brain another source of energy, which provides the brain with sufficient supplies of glutamic acid and glutamate for processing GABA. This process helps balance and reduces the excess firing of neurons, leading to better mental focus. Moreover, studies show that increased production of GABA reduces anxiety and stress, which also helps improve mental clarity.

Release Energy for Healing

Have you ever worked for more than 8 to 10 hours a day with a massive project, especially when the boss asks you to do something beyond your pay grade or job title? Then you have a precise idea how your body feels when it has to process the food you eat 24 hours a day, 7 days a week.

You put your body under duress. Similar to the way you cope with a considerable workload, your body will deal. It must cope and make important decisions. It attends to the most urgent and important tasks first, setting aside matters that can wait for another day. The more you stuff yourself with food, the more you put it into overwork, whether it is ready or not to take on a new job. Eventually, it cannot keep up, and you experience various health problems. Just like a mean boss dumping another stack of papers to process when you still have 3 tall piles on your desk.

You can take a vacation when you are feeling weary, under-appreciated, and overworked. Your body on the other hand, rarely gets a break, mainly when you eat almost every hour of the day.

Fasting is giving your body its well-deserved vacation from constant feeding. When you eat, the digestive system utilizes up to 65 percent of the energy. Digestion, along with all the other process it needs for the day takes a lot of energy. At the end of the day, your body does not have enough fuel for other essential tasks.

During intermittent fasting, your body diverts energy towards recuperation and healing. Moreover, when you fast, your body undergoes detoxification, efficiently eliminating metabolic wastes naturally produced by healthy cells, as well as foreign toxins. Your system can also spend more fuel on the cell, tissue, and organ repairs instead of just eliminating the byproducts of eating.

Fasting will allow your body to catch up on the critical tasks that it has put aside. During this period, the system will finally be able to handle all the toxins, cleaning the excess toxins from the tissues, thus, creating a stage or an environment for healing.

Fosters Spiritual Growth

As you continually remove heavy and unhealthy food from your diet and detoxify, your body will feel less dense and become lighter. Shedding all the excess fat during the process also makes you lighter. Moreover, fasting reduces sleep disorders and fatigues, helping you attain inner harmony and balance.

When you are healthier, your focus will shift from the worldly things and physical reality towards the aspects of your life that indeed matter instead of your health problems.

The practice of intermittent fasting also fosters discipline, which sharpens spiritual senses, mainly when you practice it together with meditation. Completing self-imposed tasks strengthens your willpower, thus, teaching you to manage your life better, particularly during stressful situations.

Reasons Why Fasting Works

Aside from people's obsession with excess fat and weight loss, there are other reasons why you need to practice intermittent fasting as often as you can, depending on your state of health. Here are few reasons why.

Relaxing

Once you are fasting, there's nothing much to worry about as you don't need to prepare something for your meal not worry about the kind of meal that will have adverse effects on your health. You can just gulp down a glass of water and start your day. Imagine when you have one meal less in a day or one whole day without the regular meals. One day spent less on preparing food is one more day to pamper yourself with a full relaxation. However, it doesn't mean, however, that when you're fasting, you will look gloomy or ash-fallen.

Most of you will probably be expecting someone less energetic or downfallen when on fasting. However, if you ask those who are into fasting, you will be surprised to know how energetic they seem while at this stage that when they are regularly eating their meal.

Lengthens Life Span

It is common knowledge that restricting calories are one of the ways of prolonging life. Hence, when you are fasting, your body is finding a way of extending your life. When you are on the intermittent diet, your body is activating the calorie restriction in response to lengthening your life. With this, you get the benefit of extended life without really experiencing real starvation. A study about alternate day intermittent fasting in mice done way back in 1945 proves that fasting indeed led to a longer lifespan.

Complement Chemo Therapy

There is this study of cancer patients that disclosed the side effects of chemotherapy. According to the study, patients who undergo fasting before the treatment experience diminished these side effects. Moreover, a study asserts that IF significantly increases the impact of chemotherapy or radiation. Further, research backs up on the alternate-day intermittent fasting, which leads to a conclusion that IF before chemotherapy session results in higher positive result rates and fewer deaths. In a comprehensive analysis of various studies of diseases and fasting, it appears that intermittent fasting does reduce not only the risk of cancer but also has a positive effect on cardiovascular diseases.

Key Takeaways:

- During intermittent fasting, your body undergoes various hormonal adaptations, including decrease insulin levels, stimulate the production of growth hormone, increase adrenaline levels, and regulate cell, hormone, and gene functions.

- The various hormonal changes your body undergoes during fasting helps boost weight loss, burn belly fat faster, repair cells, alter gene expression, relieve inflammation, develop strong heart, lengthens lifespan, and release energy for healing, as well as compliment chemotherapy.

- Aside from the positive physical effects, fasting improves your focus and mental clarity, as well as foster spiritual growth.

Chapter 3: Effectively Adapting to the Healthy Change

During caloric restriction (CR) and intermittent fasting, your body will be undergoing changes that could be 360 degrees different from your usual eating habits and the amount of food you consume every day. It will transition from a glucose-fueled system into a fat-burning machine.

The CR and IF will initiate various processes and adaptations until your body is ultimately transformed into a healthy, efficient system. Among the concerns and effects, you need to prepare for the following. Knowing what you have to deal with during fasting will ensure that you successfully adjust to these health practices.

Electrolyte Deficiency

There are misplaced concerns about CR and IF causing malnutrition. These misconceptions are just not correct. The body contains sufficient amount of stored glycogen and fat as the source of energy.

The primary concern during fasting is micronutrient deficiency. However, studies reveal that even prolonged IF do not cause malnutrition. Potassium levels may slightly decrease. However, even 2 months of continuous practice does not reduce the levels below 3.0 milliEquivalents per liter (mEq/L), even without supplements, which is just slightly below the average level of 3.5-5.0 mEq/L. Two months of continues fasting is more extended than recommended and you would not be doing this method on the IF.

On the other hand, phosphorus, calcium, and magnesium remain stable during fasting, which is presumably due to the large stores of them in the bones - about 90 percent of the body's phosphorus and calcium.

Taking a multi-vitamin supplement during CR and IF provides the body of the recommended daily micronutrient allowance. In fact, a 382-day therapeutic fast with multivitamin showed to have no detrimental effect on health. The only related result was the slight uric acid elevation, which exhibited after the hundredth day of fasting.

Uric Acid Elevation

"A study of the Retention of Uric Acid during Fasting" revealed that a 21-fasting period caused a significant increase of the concentration of uric acid in the blood, which was the result of the decreased elimination uric acid. Reduced urine volume seems to be the leading cause of the build-up, as well as the changes in metabolism and kidney functions the system undergoes during IF. The study further stated that ketosis seems to alter the oxidation and the acid-base equilibrium of the body tissues and blood that result in a uric acid increase.

To prevent and/or remedy this side effect, you must:

- Drink sufficient amount of water to dilute uric acid and help the kidneys excrete it more efficiently.

- Increase the alkalinity of the body by eating more vegetables during the feeding period. You can ass boiled beans and peas into your meals to add alkalinity and fullness taste.

- If you have high uric acid before starting fasting, then going vegan or vegetarian might be a good idea.

- Add 1/2 teaspoon baking soda in a glass of water and drink 3 times a day.

- Reduce meat because they contain high purine.

- Avoid alcoholic drinks. Drink coffee or tea instead.

- Blueberries and cherries help reduce pain due to the formation of uric acid crystals.

After-Fast Weight Gain

Gaining weight after the fasting period is normal. The added weight is mostly water weight gain, and you might acquire some fat. Short-term weight gain happens after you break your fats. Once you start eating again, you will see the added weight on your scale.

Do not worry! This gain is temporary. Stored glycogen in the body is heavily hydrated because they are bound to water. During fasting, you use the stored glycogen for energy, so you lose weight. When you enter the feeding state, you will gain water weight as your body replenishes glycogen stores. Moreover, sodium also retains water, which also adds to water weight gain.

This almost immediate additional weight is not excess fat. It is just your body getting back to normal after fasting. Moreover, restricting your calorie intake during fasting drives your body to increase stored energy or body fat for a future period with reduced calories.

Do not fret! More importantly, do not worry. Your body is still transitioning from a glucose-fueled system into a fat-burning machine. Your body will not adapt to the changes right away. But as you continue your fasting practice, your body will soon efficiently utilize fat as its source of energy and burn them. Here are tips to help your body adapt to a fat-fueled system faster.

- Avoid junk and food, alcohol, and sugar, especially during the first week of fasting. These foods provide the body with glucose that feeds fat deposits during the transition period when the body is driven to increase energy storage.

- Consume low glycemic carbohydrates, such as vegetables, legumes, beans, and whole grains. These foods are digested slower, preventing the surge of blood sugar that the body turns into fat as it seeks to replenish energy stores when you break your fast.

- Consume high-quality protein, such as seeds and nuts, legumes, beans, whole grain, low-fat dairy, fish, and meat. They decrease hunger and reduce the body's dependency on carbs for energy, as well as help promote muscle growth.

- Consume low-calorie-density food, such as whole grains and vegetables. They are high in fiber and low in calories per bite, which reduce the sugar you feed your body.

Lean Muscle Mass Loss

This issue is another crucial concern relating intermittent fasting. Does IF burn muscle? The straight answer is NO. In fact, a study revealed that during fasting, the body does not start burning muscle, it starts conserving it. Moreover, physiologic studies concluded that protein is not 'burnt' for glucose.

When the body achieves the state of ketosis, there is no need to use protein for gluconeogenesis or converting amino acids into glucose because the body metabolizes fatty acids as the source of energy. During normal conditions, the body breaks down 75 grams of protein daily. However, during fasting, this falls to about 15 to 20 grams daily. So IF actually decreases muscle breakdown.

Moreover, intermittent fasting boosts the levels of growth hormone and insulin-like growth factor I that promote muscle growth and increased muscle strength.

If you are worried about the lean muscle mass loss, then provide the body with sufficient sources of fatty acid to burn as energy.

Not Everyone Can Fast

Intermittent Fasting is not for everyone. Like other health programs, there are significant rules and exemptions.

Those Who Shouldn't Fast

If you belong to these types of people, then it is advisable for you not to fast.

- Diabetic and hypoglycemic patients
- Those who are underweight
- Those with low blood pressure
- Those with eating disorder
- Those who are under medications
- Pregnant and breastfeeding women
- Women with amenorrhea and fertility problems
- Women who are trying to get conceived
- Those with cortisol deregulation
- Those suffering from chronic stress

Consult a healthcare professional or your doctor if you are uncertain that you can fast. If you have determined that you cannot practice, you can do a cleansing diet instead to detoxify and gain many, if not all, of the benefits of fasting. Cleansing options often create the same detox effects as IF, eliminating toxins and rebuilding healthy tissue, but in a gradual manner.

Fasting for Women

There is some evidence that shows that fasting is less beneficial to women as it is for their male counterparts. It turns out that women's bodies react differently to IF than men's bodies. Females are more sensitive to the signals of hunger. Additionally, the hormones that regulate vital functions like ovulation are extremely sensitive to energy intake. Some women do just fine with intermittent fasting while others experience problems. Even short-term CR and IF can alter the hormonal pulses in some females, disrupting regular and specific cycles.

Moreover, if not done correctly, caloric restriction and intermittent fasting can cause various hormonal imbalances. When the female body senses that it is hungry, it will increase the production of hunger hormones, ghrelin, and leptin. This reaction is the body's way to protect a potential fetus, even when the woman is not pregnant.

Of course, when you are practicing CR and IF, you will ignore these hunger signals, causing the body to produce more hunger hormones, which can throw everything out of balance.

Although there are no studies conducted in humans, rat experiments revealed that intermittent fasting had some adverse effects on female rats. It developed these female rats into masculine-like, infertile, and emaciated rats while causing them to miss cycles. The ovaries shrunk and the menstrual cycles stopped while they experienced more insomnia than males. Moreover, studies show that CR and IF can aggravate eating disorders like bulimia, anorexia, and binge eating disorder.

So how do women approach caloric restriction and intermittent fasting?

Intermittent Fasting Options for Women

For women, the general guidelines for successful IF are as follows:

- Fasting should not last more than 24 hours for periods.

- Women should fast for about 12 to 16 hours only.

- Avoid fasting on consecutive days during the first 2 to 3 weeks of IF. For instance, if you are doing a 16-hour fast, do it 3 days a week instead of 7 days.

- Drink plenty of fluids during your fast, such as water, herbal tea, and bone broth.

- During fasting days, only do light exercises, such as gentle stretching, jogging, walking, and yoga.

Also, several intermittent fasting methods are suitable for women. Here are the most popular ones that you can try.

Crescendo Method

This method is the best way for women to ease into caloric restriction and intermittent fasting without disrupting hormones or shocking the body. This type does not require a female to fast a week, only for a couple of days spaced throughout the period.

For example, fasting for 12 to 16 hours every Monday, Wednesday, and Friday with an eating window of 8 to 12 hours.

The other 3 IF methods best suited for women are the 16/8 Method or the Leangains method, the Eat-Stop-Eat or 24-Hour Protocol, and the 5:2 Diet, which are all discussed in Chapter 4: Listen to the Needs of Your Body.

Stop intermittent fasting if you experience any of the following. These symptoms often indicate that you are experiencing a hormonal imbalance.

- When menstrual cycle becomes irregular or stops
- Experience problems staying or falling asleep
- Falling hair, acne breakout, and dry skin
- Having a hard time recovering from workouts
- Injuries heal slowly and getting sick more often
- The heart starts to beat irregularly or in a weird-manner

- Having mood swings

- Experiencing decreased tolerance to stress

- Feeling cold

- Digestion significantly slows down

- Less interested in sex

Key Takeaways:

- Changing your eating schedule and habit can cause some concerns, such as electrolyte deficiency, uric acid elevation, after-fast weight gain, and lean muscle loss. However, studies show that you can quickly remedy all these side effects.

- Research shows that fasting does not reduce the amount of electrolyte in the body significantly.

- Taking a multi-vitamin supplement during fasting provides the body of the recommended daily micronutrient allowance.

- Fasting can cause a slight elevation in uric acid, but you can easily prevent this from occurring by drinking plenty of water and increasing your alkalinity by eating more vegetables.

- After-fast weight gain is temporary, and most of it is water weight while you are on your regular feeding periods. As you continue fasting, your body will soon efficiently utilize fat as its source of energy and burn them, and your weight will go down eventually.

- Avoid junk and food, alcohol, and sugar, especially during the first week of fasting. Consume low glycemic carbohydrates, such as vegetables, legumes, beans, and whole grains.

- Intermittent fasting does not burn muscle. In fact, boosts the levels of growth hormone and insulin-like growth factor I that promote muscle growth and increased muscle strength. If you are worried about the lean muscle mass loss, then provide the body with sufficient sources of fatty acid to burn as energy.

- Not everyone can fast.

- Women react differently to fasting than men. For effective intermittent fasting, women need to follow a guideline that will prevent disruption of hormonal balance, which is very sensitive to hunger.

- The best fasting methods for women are the Crescendo Method, the 16/8 Method or the Leangains method, the Eat-Stop-Eat or 24-Hour Protocol, and the 5:2 Diet.

- Women should stop fasting when they experience the symptoms of hormonal imbalance.

Chapter 4: Listen to the Needs of Your Body

Fasting recalibrates your body. Practicing this weight loss method without preparation is a recipe for failure. Knowing what you'll have to deal with and choosing the best fasting method will ensure success.

Buffer Your Weight Loss and Muscle Gain Journey

Slow is the way to go, especially if you are just starting on your diet. Preparation will help your body adjust and adapt to the practice better, and help you experience less or no transition symptoms or keto flu (flu-like symptoms a person experiences as the body changes from burning glucose to fat as the primary source of energy). Planning also lessens or prevents detoxification symptoms; fasting can start a release of too many toxins into the bloodstream at one time.

Start Your Diet with a 1-Day Fruit or Juice Fast

Do this once every week until you no longer experience the detoxification symptoms or your body is ready to transition from a glucose-fueled system to fat-burning machine. An apple fruit fast is easy to begin. Start your IF the night before. Eat a light dinner. Do not overfeed yourself out of fear for the next day. On your fasting day, eat 3-4 apples as your meals and drink at least 2 quarts of water throughout the day. Cut back on caffeinated drinks on your apple fruit fast as well. If you crave for something warm during the period, drink warmed water. The next day, when you break your fast, ease into food slowly and then return to regular eating.

When your body is over the detox symptoms, try the Leangains Method (16:8 Fasting) or do a 1-day water fast. People find it easier to deal with the hunger when they slowly ease into an advanced fasting method than jumping immediately into it since the body gradually adjusts to the prospect of not feeding. You will not get too hungry right away, which is something that is difficult to deal with for some people. Eventually, your system will adjust to the no food period.

When your body has sufficiently adapted to the semi-fasting state, you can start with any of the 7 methods below. Before you proceed with your actual fasting, read them all. Weigh your options. Take an honest look at your life. How much can you sacrifice? An IF practice will create intense detoxifying and cleansing symptoms, as well as ketosis symptoms, which will require more discipline from you. How much discomfort can you take?

Do you want a fasting without a great deal of discipline? That is also very possible. Some professionals suggest avoiding extreme symptoms of detoxification by doing an easy fasting method. You can absolutely take it slower, at a pace most comfortable for you.

#1 - Leangains Method (16:8 Fasting)

Started by Martin Berkhan, Leangains Method is best recommended for dedicated fitness enthusiasts aiming to lose body fats and build muscles.

Under the Leangain method of fasting, you are allowed to eat only within 8 or 10 hours break while you are fasting for 16 hours (for men) and 14 hours (for women). During your fasting period, you are not supposed to consume calories though you are permitted to take calorie-free foods.

It is much easier to start fasting through the night until the next morning - roughly six hours after waking up. However, this needs a close maintenance feeding window else you get it harder to stick to the program while disrupting your hormones normal functioning.

The time and the kind of food that you will be eating during your feeding window largely depend on when you will be working out. On days when you are doing your workout, carbohydrates are more important than fat. However, on your rest days, you must take more fats. It is advisable to be always high on protein consumption, but it must be in proportion to your goal, gender, activity level, and body fat. Regardless of how you spend your activity, the consumption of whole and unprocessed food is preferable in choosing your calorie intake. Nonetheless, if you don't have much time for a proper meal, better grab yourself a protein bar or protein shake instead.

For most people who are into this fasting method, the highlight is the fact that in most days, meal frequency does not really matter. You can always eat anytime you want as long as it is within the eight-hour feeding window. With this, most people prefer breaking it up into three meals as it is easier to stick to it while being programmed to this eating habit.

Nonetheless, even if your eating time is flexible, Leangains fast is very specific with its guidelines regarding the kind of food that you can eat, primarily if you are working out. The rather strict guide on nutrition planning makes the program a little bit tough to adhere.

#2 - Eat Stop Eat (24-Hour Fasting)

This program involves fasting for 1 whole day (24 hours) once or twice a week. While you are fasting, you are allowed to drink calorie-free drinks. After the fasting period, you can go back to regular eating.

This method of fasting reduces overall calorie intake without putting a limit on what you eat and how often you want to eat. It is worthy to note, however, that incorporating regular workouts, including resistance training is the bottom line if your goal is a weight loss of an improved body composition.

Though it is quite hard to contemplate that you will be without food for 24 hours, still there is an excellent side of the Eat Stop Eat Fast since this option is quite flexible. You don't have to follow the rule strictly on your first day of fasting. You can go as long as you can manage and then gradually increase your fasting duration over time to give your body enough time to adjust.

It is advantageous if you start your fasting on the day when you are busy and at a time that doesn't fall on your eating schedule like lunch. Another bonus is that there are no forbidden foods, no restrictions on your diet, and no calorie counting. Even the quantity of your food intake is never an issue here. However, you must know how to moderate your eating like you can eat a slice of the cake but not the whole piece.

The long hours of Eat Stop Eat Fast prove to be challenging to some people, especially for starters. While your body is still adjusting, you can feel some symptoms like fatigue, weakness, headache or dizziness, and cranky. All these will tempt you to put a break to your fasting. However, these symptoms diminish over time while it takes a lot of self-control on your part to overcome all those negative feelings.

#3 - The Warrior Diet (20/4 Diet)

This method, which is inspired by the eating habits of warriors in the olden days, allows you fast for 20 hours every day and then eat one large meal in the evening. It is crucial to eat a quality meal rather than getting a hefty one while on your feeding period. Nonetheless, you are allowed mild consumption during the day like a few servings of raw fruits and veggies, or a few servings of protein shakes if you feel like needing it. Some warrior dieters question this option based on the logic that if you exercise this perk, then it's no longer a real fast.

This method of intermittent fasting is supposed to promote alertness, stimulates fat burning, and boost energy while maximizing the fight or flight reaction of the sympathetic nervous system. The four hours feeding state is aimed towards maximizing the ability of the parasympathetic nervous system to help the body to recuperate. Likewise, it promotes calmness, relaxation, and digestion as it helps the body generate hormones and burn fat in the daytime. Further, the order in which you eat specific food groups also matters. According to this method, you should start with vegetables, fats, and proteins. If you are still not satiated, only then will you take in some carbohydrates.

Many prefer this method of intermittent fasting as this option allows you to eat a few small meals or snacks, which can help you get through your fasting period. Many testified to have gained an increase in energy level and fat loss while on this diet.

It may be better to have a few snacks than going without any food for more than 20 hours. Still, to have strict guidelines of what needs to be eaten and when to eat them proves challenging in the long run. Also, eating one main meal at night as according to the guidelines is not easy, especially for folks who prefer minimal intake in the later part of the day.

#4 – Fat Loss Forever

The Fat Loss Forever method is a hybrid of the three practices – Eat Stop Eat, the Warrior Diet, and the Leangains as you combine them all into one single plan. You are also allowed one cheat day for each week and then follow it up by a 36-hour fast. The remainder of the one-week cycle is then split up between the different fasting methods.

In this method, it is recommended that you save the most extended fast on days when you are at your most active level. The practice allows you to focus on your productivity that on your hunger. Integrated into this intermittent fasting are training programs, free weights, and body weights, which are geared towards helping trainees maximize fat loss efficiently.

Founders of this program, John Romaniello, and Dan Go believe that everyone is practically fasting every day and these are times when we aren't eating anything and on an irregular schedule which is why we can't reap the benefit of intermittent fasting. Under the Fat Loss Forever method, there is a seven-day schedule for fasting, which helps your body get used to a structured timetable. It also includes a full-fledged cheat day, which makes the program preferable to many.

Conversely, you will have a hard time handling the cheat days because the plan is too specific and the schedule of fasting or feeding varies from day to day making it confusing to follow. If you are the type who would find it hard to quickly switch from indulging in moderation and then turning it off when it's time to change to fasting, then this program may not work well with you.

#5 - UpDayDownDay (Alternate-Day Fasting)

The easiest of all the intermittent fasting methods, the Alternate-Day Fasting or the UpDayDownDay method allows you have a minimal amount of food intake in one day and then resort back to normal eating the next day. The practice aims to lower down your calorie intake level by 1/5 of the required normal calorie intake during the day of fasting. Let's say, the regular level of calorie for men is 2,500 and for women is 2,000, in a fasting or down day, the level must be brought down to 500 for men and 400 for women.

To make it easier for you during the "down" period, opt for a meal replacement like protein shakes. You can choose your shakes to be fortified with essential nutrients, and you can take sips of your shakes throughout the day rather than opt for small meals. However, take note that meal replacements like these shakes are advisable only during the first two weeks of your fasting and you are encouraged to eat real meals on your next "down" days. Resort back to regular eating in the next days.

If you are doing some workout regimen, keep your workout days on normal-calorie days as it would be hard for you to hit the gym during low-calorie days.

As this option is all about weight loss, it works perfectly for you if your goal is towards losing weight. People who cut on their calories by 20-25 percent on the average witness a loss of approximately 2 and a half pounds every week as reported on the internet.

This method of intermittent fasting is easy to follow, and there's always a tendency for you to overindulge on it during the regular day. The trick here to stay aligned is by planning and preparing your meal ahead of time, so you don't have to indulge yourself in an eat-all-you-can or drive-thru food once you're up for the feasting.

#6 –Fast Diet (5:2 Fasting)

The Fast Diet method of intermittent fasting is also known as 5:2. As the name itself implies, you have to undergo 2 days of fasting and 5 days of regular eating within a week cycle. On your ordinary days, you won't be worrying about your calorie intake, but on the rest of the week (2 days fast days), you need to reduce your calories, e.g., 500 for women and 600 for men. With these 2 days of your choice every week, it is easier to comply with this kind of health regimen though it could take longer losing weight this way compared to the rest of intermittent fasting methods.

#7 – Daniel Fast

The Daniel Fast is a 28-day fast that combines spiritual belief and nutrition through the unlimited intake of whole, non-processed foods. This method of fasting is popular among Christian believers as it is based on the Biblical foundation as described in the Book of Daniel. (Daniel 1-10). Rather than restricting calorie intake or focusing on weight loss, Daniel Fast limits the type of food consumed to increase the quality of nutrient intake.

Although more of a religious orientation, scientific research supports the Daniel Fast. According to the T. Collin Campbell Center for Nutrition Studies, researchers reveal that those people with cardiovascular disease or metabolic dysfunction experienced an improvement when they implemented the dietary habits of the fast.

Key Takeaways:

- Knowing what you will encounter during intermittent fasting, as well as choosing the best fasting method for your lifestyle will ensure success.

- Slow is the best way to go if you are new to fasting. Buffer your journey to prevent and lessen detoxification and keto-flu symptoms.

- You can slowly ease into fasting by doing a -Day Fruit or Juice Fast, and then try the Leangains Method (16:8 Fasting) or do a 1-day water fast for a period.

- When your body has eventually adjusted to the fasting state, choose the best fasting method that is most comfortable for you, which includes Leangains Method (16:8 Fasting), Eat Stop Eat (24-Hour Fasting), The Warrior Diet (20/4 Diet), Fat Loss Forever, UpDayDownDay (Alternate-Day Fasting), Fast Diet (5:2 Fasting), and Daniel Fast.

Chapter 5: Successfully Transitioning into a Healthier You

Intermittent fasting and caloric restriction is a healthy change. During your transition, you will definitely experience hard days. Here are some tips that will make the journey easier.

Prepare for the Detoxification and Ketosis Symptoms

Unless fasting is a regular part of your health routine, you will experience, or many symptoms as your body can concentrate on removing metabolic waste and adjust to become a fat-burning machine from a glucose-fueled system.

Among the many symptoms of fasting, here are the most common ones, along with how you can efficiently deal with them.

Disrupted Sleep Patterns and Fatigue

Fasting stimulates purging of toxins that require more significant workload than typical so that you will feel more tired than usual. It will take at least 3 days for your body to overcome hunger and cravings from old habits and food. Because fasting is limited or complete abstinence of food, except water, it is a great idea to start your practice during the days when you can rest.

Take naps whenever you can and get to bed by 10 pm, making sure to get 8 hours of sleep every night. Your body works more efficiently at cleansing and repairing itself while you are sleeping. Stick to moderate or light exercise routines. Avoid stress, whether mental, emotional, or physical because they are counterproductive to your fasting.

Headache

Headaches usually happen because you are ditching some bad habits during fasting, such as cutting out processed food and sugar, smoking, caffeine, and alcoholic drinks, which creates withdrawal, causing headaches.

You may also experience dehydration during your fasting period, which also causes headaches. Drink plenty of water, a minimum of about 8 to 10 full glasses of filtered water a day.

Nausea

Changing your lifestyle and diet along with choosing healthier food may cause slight nausea. The best way to avoid this symptom is through proper hydration. Nausea usually will usually pass after a couple of days.

If your symptom advances to vomiting, then your body may be detoxifying too quickly. Your system may try to expel toxins faster than it can eliminate. The best thing to do when this occurs is to change your fasting method.

Detoxification symptoms may progress to ketosis symptoms, including flu-like symptoms, rash, and very rarely vomiting.

Cravings and Hunger

You will also experience hunger, but this will disappear in 1 to 2 days during fasting. Moreover, you will be eliminating a lot of food and drinks that your body consumes typically, such as processed food and sugar, smoking, caffeine, and alcoholic beverages. Reducing or eliminating them will most definitely trigger cravings to those areas you have removed and changed. This symptom will continue longer than hunger. When they flare up, drinking water will decrease these symptoms.

Stay Hydrated

Water will help you keep going while you are in your fasting period. It also helps you burn fats and boost your metabolism.

Prefer Overnight Fasting

When most of your fasting hours occur during the night, it is easier for you to get through it. While you hibernate, you won't be thinking of hunger and avoid food cravings.

Transform Your Thinking Process

When you're thinking of fasting as a form of depriving you of food, the more you will crave for it. But if you think of it as just a form of taking a break from eating, the lesser you will feel the pangs of hunger. Therefore, controlling your mindset can help you get through more comfortable with your fasting.

Start When You're Busy

It's better to start your fasting when you're loaded with activities as this will help your mind stay away from thinking about food. When we are thinking about IF, the idea alone will send us thinking more about food.

Hit the Gym

Mixing workout with intermittent fasting will help you optimize the result. Your exercise does not need to be hardcore. Stick with something easy and straightforward like the full-body strength routine. You can do this 2-3 times a week.

Now that you have a clear overview of what's gone trending in health and fitness programs, particularly in intermittent fasting as you have learned all about its drawbacks and benefits, you are free to choose what plan is best for you. While all of them demonstrate to be effective, you must consider your lifestyle while selecting the best option for you to get the best benefit from it.

Lastly, you have to keep in mind that intermittent fasting is never a diet and therefore works well with nearly all kinds of eating program. Meaning, you can get into intermittent fasting whatever your preferences and nutritional restrictions are. You can be a Paleo diet fanatic, a strict follower of low carb diet, a hardcore supporter of vegan, Ketogenic, low-fat or any other kind of nutritional plan, and you can easily integrate them with intermittent fasting. Intermittent fasting is a dietary lifestyle that aids you in your goal towards obtaining a healthy, lean, and strong body.

Key Takeaways:

- During your transition from a sugar-fueled system into a fat-burning machine, you will encounter some side effects

- You need to prepare for detoxification and keto-flu symptoms, including disrupted sleep patterns and fatigue, headaches, nausea, and cravings and hunger.

- You can easily prevent and remedy these side effects by staying hydrated, preferring overnight fasting, transforming your thinking process, starting your fast on busy days, and hitting the gym.

Conclusion

Upon reaching the end of your reading of this book, you have enough knowledge and probably have experienced some methods of intermittent fasting. We are hoping that this book has guided you through your decision of what program is best for you depending on several factors. Each one of the readers may have plans of undertaking intermittent fasting with different goals in mind. However, this book had focused primarily on your achieving a successful weight loss while building a healthier and leaner body while generating muscle mass.

Now that we have established that intermittent fasting is the best, quickest, and easiest way to lose weight and build a leaner structure, we are advocating for its long-term practice and execution. Make intermittent a lifetime habit, not just a fad or fashion that you use while it is popular.

Getting into the habit of intermittent fasting will give you long-lasting benefits like a healthy body and integrating it into your lifestyle will secure you away from many health risks associated with deadly illnesses.

Final Words

Thank you again for purchasing this book! I really hope this book is able to help you.

The next step is for you to **join our email newsletter** to receive updates on any upcoming new book releases or promotions. You can sign-up for free and as a bonus, you will also receive our "*7 Fitness Mistakes You Don't Know You're Making*" book! This bonus book breaks down many of the most common fitness mistakes and will demystify many of the complexities and science of getting into shape. Having all this fitness knowledge and science organized into an actionable step-by-step book will help you get started in the right direction in your fitness journey! To join our free email newsletter and grab your free book, please visit the link and signup: **www.hmwpublishing.com/gift**

Finally, if you enjoyed this book, then I would like to ask you for a favour, would you be kind enough to leave a review for this book? It would be greatly appreciated!

Thank you and good luck in your journey!

About the Co-Author

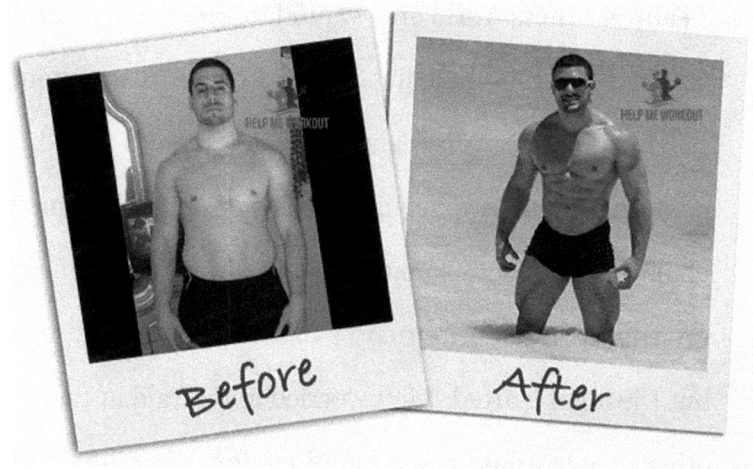

My name is George Kaplo; I'm a certified personal trainer from Montreal, Canada. I'll start off by saying I'm not the biggest guy you will ever meet and this has never really been my goal. In fact, I started working out to overcome my biggest insecurity when I was younger, which was my self-confidence. This was due to my height measuring only 5 foot 5 inches (168cm), it pushed me down to attempt anything I ever wanted to achieve in life. You may be going through some challenges right now, or you may simply want to get fit, and I can certainly relate.

For me personally, I was always kind of interested in the health & fitness world and wanted to gain some muscle due to the numerous bullying in my teenage years about my height and my overweight body. I figured I couldn't do anything about my height, but I sure can do something about how my body looked like. This was the beginning of my transformation journey. I had no idea where to start, but I just got started. I felt worried and afraid at times that other people would make fun of me for doing the exercises the wrong way. I always wished I had a friend that was next to me who was knowledgeable enough to help me get started and "show me the ropes."

After a lot of work, studying and countless trial and errors. Some people began to notice how I was getting more fit and how I was starting to form a keen interest in the topic. This led many friends and new faces to come to me and ask me for fitness advice. At first, it seemed odd when people asked me to help them get in shape. But what kept me going is when they started to see changes in their own body and told me it's the first time that they saw real results!

From there, more people kept coming to me, and it made me realize after so much reading and studying in this field that it did help me but it also allowed me to help others. I'm now a fully certified personal trainer and have trained numerous clients to date who have achieved amazing results.

Today, my brother Alex Kaplo (also a Certified Personal Trainer) and I own & operate this publishing venture, where we bring passionate and expert authors to write about health and fitness topics. We also run an online fitness website "HelpMeWorkout.com" and I would love to connect with by inviting you to visit the website on the following page and signing up to our e-mail newsletter (you will even get a free book).

Last but not least, if you are in the position I was once in and you want some guidance, don't hesitate and ask... I'll be there to help you out!

Your friend and coach,

George Kaplo
Certified Personal Trainer

Get another book for Free

I want to thank you for purchasing this book and offer you another book (just as long and valuable as this book), "Health & Fitness Mistakes You Don't Know You're Making", completely free.

Visit the link below to signup and receive it:

www.hmwpublishing.com/gift

In this book, I will break down the most common health & fitness mistakes, you are probably committing right now, and I will reveal how you can easily get in the best shape of your life!

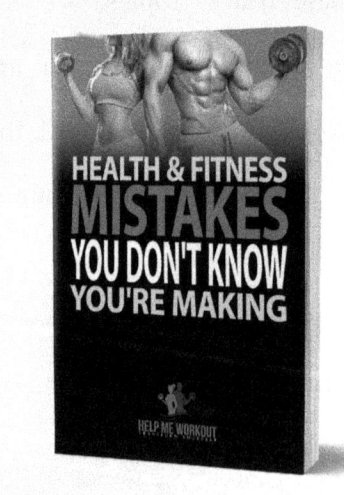

In addition to this valuable gift, you will also have an opportunity to get our new books for free, enter giveaways, and receive other valuable emails from me. Again, visit the link to sign up:

www.hmwpublishing.com/gift

Copyright 2017 by HMW Publishing - All Rights Reserved.

This document by HMW Publishing owned by the A&G Direct Inc company, is geared towards providing exact and reliable information in regards to the topic and issue covered. The publication is sold with the idea that the publisher is not required to render accounting, officially permitted, or otherwise, qualified services. If advice is necessary, legal or professional, a practiced individual in the profession should be ordered.

From a Declaration of Principles which was accepted and approved equally by a Committee of the American Bar Association and a Committee of Publishers and Associations.

In no way is it legal to reproduce, duplicate, or transmit any part of this document in either electronic means or in printed format. Recording of this publication is strictly prohibited, and any storage of this document is not allowed unless with written permission from the publisher. All rights reserved.

The information provided herein is stated to be truthful and consistent, in that any liability, in terms of inattention or otherwise, by any usage or abuse of any policies, processes, or directions contained within is the solitary and utter responsibility of the recipient reader. Under no circumstances will any legal responsibility or blame be held against the publisher for any reparation, damages, or monetary loss due to the information herein, either directly or indirectly.

The information herein is offered for informational purposes solely, and is universal as so. The presentation of the information is without contract or any type of guarantee assurance.

The trademarks that are used are without any consent, and the publication of the trademark is without permission or backing by the trademark owner. All trademarks and brands within this book are for clarifying purposes only and are the owned by the owners themselves, not affiliated with this document.

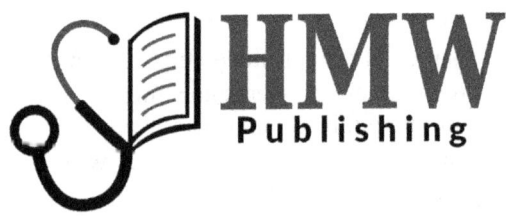

For more great books visit:

HMWPublishing.com

www.ingramcontent.com/pod-product-compliance
Lightning Source LLC
Chambersburg PA
CBHW071118030426
42336CB00013BA/2133